A note from the author

This book is not intended to change a person's way of eating, every person on this planet has the right to eat whatever they want without being judged. "Simply Rawlicious" is a book that explores the health benefits attained from eating a Raw Vegan Diet.

If after reading this book you decide to follow the Raw Vegan Diet, would suggest first that you consult your doctor before making any changes to your diet. This book is not intended as a cure for any health issues you may have.

This book is based on my personal experience being vegan. I strongly believe that one can live a long, healthy and happy life eating raw vegan food.

GO RAW!

Anthony Whitelaw

Dedication page

This book is dedicated to the following:

My wife and children for all of your love and support

My parents whom I love very much

My daughter Taliya whom I love and miss very much

My big sister for teaching me how to be strong at an early age

To everyone who partakes in the preservation of life, our planet and animal life by living a vegetarian/raw vegan plant based lifestyle.

Thank You.

Famous quotes

"We choose to eat meat and have therefore built slaughter houses for the animals and hospitals for us." – Akbarral Jetha

"A dead cow lying in the pasture is recognized as a rotting corpse, but the same carcass hung in a butcher shop passes as food."

"The love for all living creatures is the noble attribute of man." – Charles Darwin

"Nothing will benefit human health and increase chances for survival of life on earth as much as the evolution to a vegetarian diet." – Albert Einstein

"Until we stop harming all other living beings, we are all savages." – Thomas Edison

Table of Contents

Introduction to Raw foods

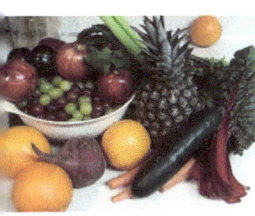

Anytime you read a magazine, surf the internet, or read the newspaper one thing is for sure – we are concerned about our health. There are several different ways to achieve a better state of health. You can make diet and lifestyle changes that result in you reaching your goals. But unfortunately, we often turn to fad diets and extreme exercising in order to achieve what we believe to be a normal state of health.

Well, doing things that are extreme are not necessarily good for you. The body is a very complex machine. It takes the right nutrients in order for the body to perform optimally. Our modern diets are depleted in a lot of these nutrients and it makes it difficult to achieve the level of health that we really want. Even a diet that is healthy by certain standards may not contain all we need. That is, unless, we consume a high amount of raw foods in order to make up for it.

In my opinion the best way to live a healthy lifestyle is to make the switch and eat a diet made up of mainly raw foods. This includes any food that is in its uncooked state. Because raw foods contain a high amount of nutrients, especially if the raw foods are also organic, it can help clear up certain health problems like obesity and heart disease and cause you to live a life that is filled with energy and free of disease.

Chapter 1

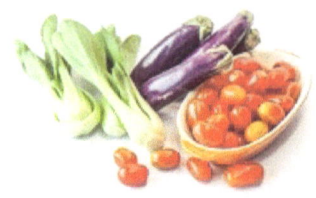

What is Vegan?

It used to be that anyone who was a vegetarian or vegan was considered a little "weird" and I suppose there are still some parts of the country that would think that way (especially in cattle country, I would guess). But more and more people are making the switch to a vegan diet.

For those of you who aren't sure what the term vegan means, it is this: Vegans, don't eat (or wear) any animal by products at all. No eggs, milk or cheese.

There are a lot of reasons people choose to become a vegan. Sometimes it's because of health issues. Cutting meat out of your diet has been shown to help lower cholesterol levels. Since meat tends to have quite a bit of saturated fat and cholesterol, even cutting back on meat may make a fairly large and positive change in your weight and cholesterol levels.

The Raw Vegan lifestyle consists of consuming non-dairy food in its unprocessed, natural form. That means eating fruits, vegetables, legumes, seeds and nuts in their organic, uncooked and unprocessed form. It also excludes all food and products of animal origin and food that is cooked at a temperature above 48 degrees Celsius, 118 degrees ahrenheit. Raw foodists believe that food cooked above this emperature will kill its nutritional value and enzymes the body needs o assist in the digestion of food.

By cooking, frying and peeling our food we take out needed nutrients our bodies need to stay healthy. Most of us were raised peeling an apple before eating it not realizing that we just peeled away ots of nutrients from that apple.

You may have heard some people use the term **"living foods"** while talking about raw foods. Is there a difference? Of course, both contain enzymes however foods like nuts need the enzymes to be activated which is done by what is called sprouting. Sprouting is when you soak nuts for example in water anywhere from 12 to 24 hours, this makes the enzyme content much higher thus making the food a living food. Living foods may include certain sprouts, fruits, vegetables, nuts and seeds. Sprouting makes assimilation of nutrition easy for the body and it does not require a lot of energy for digestion.

Chapter 2

The Basics

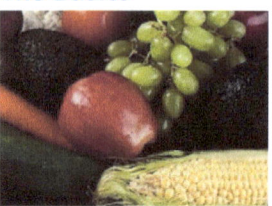

Below is a list of things to keep in mind as you make the switch o
think about making that change.

- Eating organic food is another way to increase the benefits of the Raw Vegan diet. This is because organic food is much higher in nutrients.

- If you want to eat a pure Raw Vegan diet nothing should be cooked.

- Eating a Raw Vegan diet will save you time in the kitchen because you won't need to prepare long elaborate meals.

If followed correctly and with the right mindset the Raw Vegan lifestyle can benefit your life and your health considerably. And if you are looking to make the switch, it is easy to follow especially if you choose the vegan route.

If you are undecided, try following it for a month to see if it is something that you can stick to. If it isn't, consider scaling back on you percentage. Even if you are unwilling to give up cooked foods entirely, even a diet of 80% raw foods can be beneficial. This is because you will still be getting the benefit of the extra enzymes and the nutrients that are present in raw foods.

Chapter 3

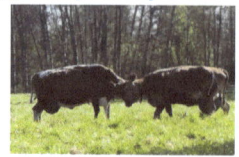

When people think of protein, the word meat usually springs to mind. We were always told that a steak or chicken or pork chop was the best source, but animal proteins have some inherent problems. First off, eating meat raw can be downright hazardous! Animal meats can contain bacteria and other pathogens that are dangerous, and even lethal if left untreated. As a result, cooking is required. However, this process contains difficulties as well. Proteins are assemblies of amino acids. When they are heated, links form between these acids, and they resist the efforts of digestive enzymes to break them down. When this happens, the body cannot absorb the proteins, and they thus become waste. This thus has two negative effects on your body: first, you are deprived of the proteins you need, and your body is now saddled with material that must be eliminated. The proteins can accumulate in the lower intestine, and become a breeding ground for bacteria and other harmful organisms. This is why I suggest an occasional colon flush to get rid of all of those harmful bacteria.

This is where eating vegetable proteins is preferable, and eating them raw is the best means of assuring you're getting the full benefits of the proteins. Now, some vegetables – most notably Lima beans and soybeans have some natural toxins in them that are made safe by cooking, but they are the exception as opposed to the rule. By and large, cooking of any sort damages the nutritional benefits of most fruits and vegetables; the higher the temperatures, the more detrimental the effects. This is yet another reason to only steam vegetables – if you insist on cooking them at all, or maybe lightly boiling or grilling them.

The key benefit of many fruits and vegetables is that they can be safely ingested when raw. Normally, just washing them is enough, and then you can eat them as-is. In doing so, you get the full benefit of their amino acids.

Along these same lines, vitamins are very susceptible to damage by heat. Vitamins such as thiamin, Vitamin B, C, and others loose much of their potency during the baking process. Others, the lipid soluble ones like K, E, D, and A suffers nearly a fifty percent drop in their effectiveness. For some vitamins, it has to do with the pH of the compound they are contained in. As an example, thiamin does not do well in anything with a pH higher than six. Above that level, nearly all of that vitamin breaks down, and is rendered useless to your health. That is why baked goods such as crackers and cookies have essentially no thiamin.

Beyond that, there's also the argument for eating fresh fruits and vegetables, as opposed to canned. The canning process has been shown to be very damaging to vitamins such as B6.

Heat is also the enemy of fats. If cooked at too high a temperature, the lipids are changed, and they bond with the walls of the body's cells. This causes blockage for the cell, and makes it difficult to function properly. Over time, this can boost your risk of heart disease and cancer.

Of all the forms of cooking, deep-frying has got to be the worst! Any food deep-fried: chicken, French fries, and so forth have a huge amount of these damaging lipids, given the popularity of such foods in the United States, its little wonder that cancer, diabetes, obesity and heart disease are so common.

Chapter 4

The raw Vegan diet is becoming very popular these days. People who support the raw Vegan diet as a healthy lifestyle argue that foods in their natural state contain the optimum balance of enzymes, vitamins and minerals that our bodies need. They argue that the enzymes contained in raw food and which are killed off by cooking, will help people to digest their food more fully and derive more nutritional value from it. That places less stress on the body to produce its own digestive enzymes.

Raw Vegans also believe that cooking our food destroys their natural vitamins and minerals and that food takes longer to digest in his cooked, unnatural state. The cooked food therefore hangs around longer in the colon while the body attempts to digest it. The proteins, carbohydrates and fats which have not been fully digested therefore become waste products. These waste products slow down the food's transit through the colon, causing constipation, bloating, stomach cancer etc, while the fats tend to clog up the arteries.

Basically, a raw food diet makes your whole digestion process a lot more efficient. It delivers more of the essential vitamins and nutrients which our bodies need and leaves behind fewer waste products which can become harmful to our bodies.

The health benefits of the raw food diet include an increase in energy as your body is maximizing the amount of nutrients it actually gets where it needs it; plus the body has to work less in order to process the raw food.

Because the Raw Vegan diet is high in fiber your digestive system will work more efficiently. Food will pass through the colon more quickly and waste will be expelled regularly.

Because of poor diet and lack of exercise heart disease is a big problem in our modern society. The Raw Vegan diet contains a higher content of nutrients and enzymes than normal so because of this, heart disease risk goes down dramatically.

Since a raw foods diet is detoxifying and not harmful, the skin will clear up, your hair will become shinier and the nails will become stronger. You will definitely lose weight while eating raw. This may be because raw foods are naturally low in fat and calories. Also, eating certain raw foods such as celery actually burns more calories to digest than the actual food, meaning that it has negative calories.

All in all, you can see that eating a diet that is comprised of raw fruits and vegetables is great for your health.

Chapter 5

All about the enzymes

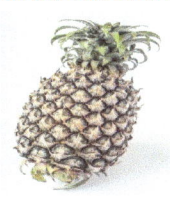

No matter what our bodies need to digest, enzymes play a crucial part of that process and as we age our bodies may not be producing all of the enzymes we need. Not only that, but the modern diet is traditionally hard on the digestive system and it has to work overtime to digest the foods we eat. This means it needs to work hard to produce all of the enzymes needed.

This is where raw foods come in. Raw foods already come equipped with enzymes in them and they help relieve the pressure on our digestive systems. This in turn helps the digestive system work at an optimum level. It also helps the body conserve enzymes and prevents some of the drastic slow-down that the digestive system experience as we age.

Chapter 6

Heat - the enemy of nutrients

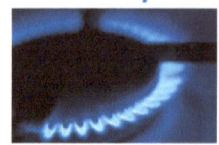

The best types of cooking are steaming, boiling, and grilling. The reason is that they generally accomplish one of the following: the food isn't cooked at an overly high temperature, and they aren't cooked for long. It may surprise you to know this, but all it takes is cooking a food at a temperature higher than 117 (Fahrenheit) for more than three minutes, and the negative impacts begin. Here are just some of the things that happen to foods kept at high temperatures for a long time:

The amino acids in the proteins essentially coagulate! They form strong links between the acid chains, and become very difficult for your body to digest. The carbohydrates become caramelized, and are rendered virtually useless to your body. This is much like the process of baking bread when the crust forms. In the old days, we were always told that the best nutrients were in the crust, and that we should eat it. Well, turns out that old wives tale was wrong. Other than a bit of roughage, the crust does you no good. And this is what high temperature and a long cooking time does to all carbohydrates!

Then there are the fats. Your body needs fats for metabolism and the construction of new cells. Excess fats are either metabolized or stored in the body. This is how we get the so-called spare tire and love handles. The thing is, too much heat and time breaks down with lipids in the fats, and you end up getting a host of cancer-causing chemicals in your body. Things with fancy names like acrolein, nitrosamines, and benzopyrene, which is one of the worst of the cancer chemicals known to exist!

Many people eat vegetables for the fiber, which is very good for you. Here again, the cellulose in fiber is severely damaged by heat. Many of its vitamins and minerals are destroyed, and the fiber's effectiveness in helping to keep your colon clear is reduced substantially.

As if that isn't bad enough; it's been found that some pesticides – while destroyed by cooking are still dangerous. The heat causes their molecules to form new compounds, which are just as bad for us to be eating! So, rather than fill up your diet with a lot of baked goods, look into the raw foods. The health benefits are innumerable.

When you make the choice to go raw you are keeping your body's enzyme reserves intact and also preventing the food from losing vital nutrients, vitamins, and minerals. Keeping these things present in food is an important part of being healthy.

Chapter 7

Getting enough protein

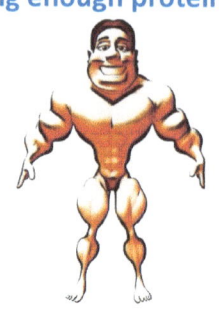

You can't write a book and not address the biggest question every Raw Vegan will hear and that is where do you get your protein from? First let me start off saying that a vegan not getting enough protein in their diet is a big misconception and nothing can be further from the truth. When you cook that steak or burger for dinner you are not consuming the amount of protein you think you are, in fact, you are actually getting less. As previously stated when you consume cooked food you are killing enzymes and amino acids that make up protein thus leaving you with nothing but empty calories along with other things that are bad for the body. When those empty calories sit in your colon because of poor digestion, bacteria will soon grow inside your colon thus causing colon cancer and other illnesses.

Even though animal products are considered superior sources of protein, there are plenty of great protein sources in the plant kingdom. The goal is to make sure you get enough of it and it is easier than you think. Even fruits and vegetables have protein, so you will end up with more than enough protein. Just make sure to have a few servings a day of some of these protein rich foods:

- Legumes such as lentils. Make sure to pair these with a grain to make for a complete protein.

- Raw nuts and seeds (not roasted)

- Grains, especially protein rich ones like quinoa

Below are examples of how many grams of protein you can get from a plant based diet:

Vegetables

1 cup of Spinach = 5 grams (you can use in salads or smoothies)

1 avocado = 10 grams

1 cup of broccoli = 5 grams

Nuts and seeds

1 oz. sesame seeds = 6.5 grams

1 oz. pistachios = 5.8 grams

2 oz. (1/4 cup) walnuts = 5 grams

2 tbsp. almonds = 4 grams

Non-dairy milk

Soy or almond. 1 cup alone will give you 7-9 grams of protein.

Grains

1 cup quinoa = 9 grams

1 cup wheat gluten (Seitan) = 52 grams (I recommend not eating a lot of it because of the amount of sodium intake).

There are also vegan protein powders you can use for protein shakes or smoothies for example, you can use 30 grams of hemp powder in your shake or smoothie and that will give you 11 grams of protein. Just make sure to use the raw protein powder. So you see how easy it is to get plenty of protein from a plant based diet and this is just a small example. Do your research and you will see that there are plenty of ways to get your protein other than consuming meat.

Chapter 8

Milk does the body bad

As stated previously vegans do not consume any dairy products and all for good reason. I'm sure you have seen the countless commercials the dairy industry has shot using celebrities wearing the milk mustache, if you take a closer look at cow's milk and what's in it you may think twice about drinking that chocolate shake or eating that cheese pizza made with milk.

Recombinant bovine growth hormone or rbgh for short is a genetically artificial hormone injected into dairy cows to make them produce 10% more milk than usual. We humans have in our blood a hormone called igf and when we consume dairy from a cow that has been injected with the rbgh hormone it raises the igf hormone in our blood which in turn causes breast, prostate and testicular cancer. Also studies have shown that cow's milk is full of pus, antibiotics, hormones, blood and who knows what else.

In my opinion people don't listen to their body. I hear people everywhere I go saying that they are lactose intolerant meaning they can't drink milk because it makes their stomach hurt but you still see them eating a cheeseburger and a milkshake. I was one of those people. Your stomach hurting should be enough to let you know that dairy is bad for you.

The good news is that now you can still enjoy that milkshake and that cheese pizza because of the many new vegan products that are available. Now I will be the first to admit that there may be one or two that you won't like but don't stop trying just because of one product. I will name a couple of non-dairy products that I think are delicious and believe you will agree. For cheese lovers like myself I love this vegan cheese called Daiya cheese. They make cheddar and mozzarella vegan cheese and it melts great if you want to make a pizza. There is also a vegan mayonnaise called Vegenaise that taste great. For milk lovers there are soy based milks and almond milk (my favorite) for those who avoid soy. There are also tons of dairy-free ice creams that you can enjoy and again just do your research.

Chapter 9

Macronutrients vs Micronutrients

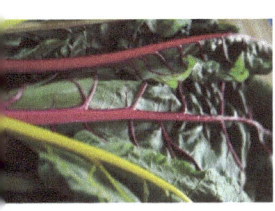

There are two types of nutrients: Macronutrients and Micronutrients. A diet that contains processed foods, meat and dairy also contains Macronutrients. When you consume too many macronutrients which contain too much fat, carbohydrates and too much protein then you become overweight and you speed up the aging process. You also promote strokes and heart attacks.

A plant based diet that includes fruits and vegetables without meat and dairy contain micronutrients. Micronutrients do not contain calories instead, they contain vitamins and minerals and phytochemicals which is why you rarely see an overweight vegan or a vegan suffering from heart attacks, strokes, diabetes etc.

Chapter 10

Tips for balancing the raw vegan diet

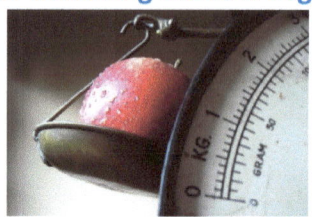

The raw foods diet is already rich in vitamins, minerals, and other nutrients so now all you need to do is put these things in the right balance. Here are some basic guidelines to follow to get you started.

• Eat a wide variety of fresh fruits and vegetables, preferably organic. You may even want to experiment with growing your own.

• Be sure to incorporate plenty of plant based protein rich foods into your diet.

• Eat a wide variety of acceptable grains.

• Drink plenty of water. Filtered or spring water is best unless you completely trust your water source.

In the beginning you can keep a food journal to help plan your menus. This is a good way to help you make sure that you are getting he right nutrients in the right proportions. If you plan your meals in advance, it will increase the likelihood that the food will be as healthy as possible.

Chapter 11

Equipment you will need

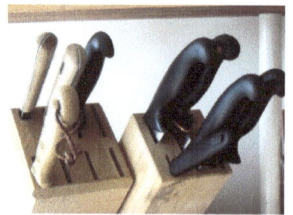

When you decide to make that transition to the raw vegan diet your kitchen will need to be stocked with the right equipment. Here are some ideas:

- If you choose to dehydrate food, of course you will need a dehydrator.

Starting off I wouldn't purchase a big expensive one, wait until you get more creative and more experience. Until then a simple one will be fine.

- A high quality juicer is a real asset. Juices can bring a lot of variety and pleasure to the diet. Choose a versatile and powerful machine that doesn't leave behind a lot of waste.

- A high powered blender like a Vitamix is a must. You will soon find out like me you can't live without it. If you own a Vitamix they are great for making smoothies, dressings, soups, the list goes on. If you do not own one I highly suggest that you purchase one.

- Standard kitchen tools like knives, bowls, and spoons are also a must have. If you make it a habit to soak beans, legumes, and grains you will also want to find some large containers with lids so that you can cover them as you soak them overnight.

Chapter 12

It gets easier

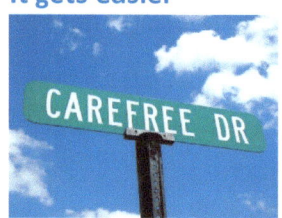

The first week will probably be the most confusing for you but don't worry, it does get easier. You can make changes gradually so you don't get overwhelmed. For example, you can set a goal to have one completely raw meal each day for the first week or so and gradually add more raw meals and snacks in the coming weeks. Don't over think things and you will be just fine.

Chapter 13

Recipes

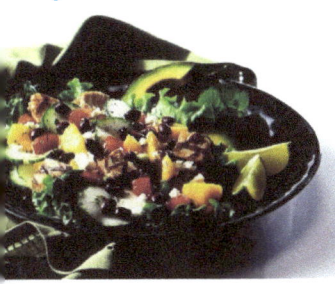

A book about the raw vegan diet would not be a book without great recipes. Here are a few to get you going.

Appetizers

Lettuce Wraps

Ingredients:

- 2 ripe avocados, pitted and mashed
- 2 tomatoes, chopped
- ½ yellow onion, diced
- 2 cloves fresh garlic, chopped
- ¼ cup fresh chopped parsley
- Kernels from one ear of fresh corn
- Juice from half a lime
- 6-8 romaine lettuce leaves (large)

Add the first seven ingredients to a large medium bowl. Mix until well combined. Place two tablespoons of the mixture in the center of each lettuce leaf. Roll the leaf up and present it on a platter.

HUMMUS

Hummus is a classic but most recipes call for canned chickpeas. Instead, buy dried chickpeas and soak them overnight or until they get soft.

Ingredients:

- 2 cups chickpeas, soaked
- 1 tablespoon water
- 1/3 cup fresh lemon juice
- 1/4 cup pitted black olives, diced

Instructions:

Combine all of the ingredients in a food processor or blender and pulse until creamy. Transfer to a serving dish and serve with crackers, bread, or whole grain pita wedges.

Smoothies

BASIC SMOOTHIE RECIPE

This is a basic smoothie recipe that can be adapted to suit your tastes. You may want to use frozen fruit to make it thicker. Smoothies also make a great dessert.

Ingredients:

- ½ cup chopped banana
- ½ cup strawberries
- 1 cup raw almond milk, raw
- Raw spinach or kale

Combine all the ingredients in a blender. Pulse until smooth and creamy.

Tropical green smoothie

2 cups of water

1 cup of grapes (green or red)

1 big handful of Spinach

1 frozen banana

1 Avocado

1/2 cup of frozen cherries

2 cups of ice

Mix all ingredients into your Vitamix , blend and enjoy!

Conclusion

This e-book is designed to give you a quick start into the world of raw foods. There are plenty of cookbooks, recipes and ideas out there that will help make your transition go smoothly.

Try to stick with it for at least a few weeks. It is important to keep a journal so you can log your progress. That way you can tell if your health is really improving or not.

Most importantly, have fun with your new lifestyle change. It is important to take charge of your health by feeding it the right foods. The raw foods diet can take you one step closer to reaching the state of health you've always dreamed of.

Thank you for your support.

Please visit www.simplyrawlicious.org

Follow us on Twitter @srawlicious

www.ingramcontent.com/pod-product-compliance
Lightning Source LLC
Chambersburg PA
CBHW050913290526
45792CB00002B/795